Preface

One of the leading news stories of 1987–88 has been the issue of surrogate motherhood that came to public attention in the much-publicized case of "Baby M." On February 3, 1988, the New Jersey Supreme Court issued a decision in this case, reversing a lower court ruling and declaring surrogate mother contracts invalid and illegal in that state.

Although this case has generally been presented by the media in a sensationalized way, much broader issues are at stake. These range from the nature of women's oppression under capitalism, to the responsibilities for child-raising, to the working-class struggle for economic justice and social progress.

The four articles in this pamphlet by *Militant* staff writer Cindy Jaquith look at these issues and the debate surrounding them. They were originally published in the April 24, May 1, and July 3, 1987, and February 19, 1988, issues of the *Militant,* a socialist newsweekly published in New York.

How 'surrogate mother' contracts exploit children and women

PUBLISHED APRIL 24, 1987

The New Jersey court case of "Baby M" reveals a brazen disregard for children. The very term "Baby M" captures the callousness with which this infant has been treated, more as an anonymous object than as a human being deserving all the protection and nurture society can offer.

By taking the child away from her mother, Mary Beth Whitehead, and by upholding a "surrogate mother" contract, Judge Harvey Sorkow has struck a blow against rights for which the working class has fought for over a century and a half.

You would never know this from the debates that raged for weeks in the courtroom and the media. Instead, a myriad of prejudices against women and working people—some falsely presented as feminist ideas—were put forward, along with a generous dose of pseudoscience and mysticism.

If we peel away each layer of the arguments presented, it becomes clear that Sorkow's March 31, 1987, ruling is reactionary and should be reversed. The child should be returned to Whitehead.

The case began when William and Elizabeth Stern went to a surrogacy agency to hire a woman to bear them a child.

Agency head Noel Keane arranged a contract between William Stern and Mary Beth Whitehead. Whitehead signed papers agreeing to be artificially inseminated with Stern's sperm, carry a pregnancy to term, and then deliver her baby to the Sterns for $10,000 plus medical expenses.

But over the course of her pregnancy and the birth of the baby in March 1986, Whitehead decided she wanted to keep her child, whom she named Sara. She informed the Sterns and said they should keep their $10,000.

The Sterns filed suit and immediately got Judge Sorkow to order Whitehead to hand her daughter over to them. The Sterns then went to Whitehead's house with five cops to seize five-week-old Sara.

Whitehead escaped with the child to Florida, but private detectives hired by the Sterns tracked them down. The detectives took Sara away and turned her over to the Sterns, who renamed her Melissa.

Judge Sorkow had no right to intervene and take Whitehead's child away. This was *not* a custody case.

The moment the Sterns asked Sorkow for a court order, he should have refused, since a surrogacy contract has no validity. There is no way a court can make it binding within the framework of the rights guaranteed by the U.S. Constitution.

In previous centuries, many working people were forced to immigrate to this country as indentured servants. They got passage in return for contracting their labor, and often that of their children, as servants for a specific time period once they arrived. If they ceased working for the person who held the contract before the time was up, they went to jail.

This practice of semislavery was outlawed through struggles of workers and farmers in the first half of the nineteenth century. Along with indentured servitude, property qualifications for voting and debtors' prisons were also abolished. So was the practice of shipping companies forcibly dragging seamen back on board if they failed to return to the ship at the end of port calls.

Today, workers cannot be forced to carry out the terms of a contract with an employer if they choose to terminate it for whatever reason. The Thirteenth Amendment to the U.S. Constitution—won by the victory of the Union in the Civil War—outlaws such contracts.

Surrogate mother contracts are similar to involuntary servitude contracts in many respects, and just as exploitative, unjust, and invalid. The woman signs a contract guaranteeing she will carry a pregnancy for someone else for nine months. According to Judge Sorkow's ruling, she is legally bound to this contract whether or not she changes her mind.

This is bad enough—but it's even worse given the nature of the rights she gives up. With the contract she signed Whitehead relinquished control of her body for nine months. She had to agree to "assume all risks" of the pregnancy, "including the risk of death." She had to agree to "abortion on demand of William Stern" if the fetus showed signs of "physiological abnormalities," determined by the doctor being paid by Stern.

Whitehead herself could not choose to have an abortion without "breaking" the contract. She also had to agree not to smoke, drink liquor, or use medications not prescribed by the Stern-paid doctor during her pregnancy.

While these conditions were imposed on Whitehead, the contract allowed Stern to terminate the agreement immediately if Whitehead had a miscarriage in the first five months. And he wouldn't have to pay her a cent.

The other side of the contract that has no validity is that Whitehead agreed *nine months beforehand* to surrender a child she planned to bear. This is completely inhumane, both to the child and mother. Under adoption law, a woman has a period of time after her baby is born to decide if she wants to put the child up for adoption, even if she concluded at some point in her pregnancy that this is what she wanted to do.

Gary Skoloff, the Sterns' lawyer, made the fantastic argument in court that surrogacy contracts are actually an advance for women's rights. "You prevent women from becoming surrogate mothers and deny them the freedom to decide . . . it's being unfairly paternalistic and it's an insult to the female population of this country," he claimed.

This argument was defended by Jan Sutton, spokeswoman for a group called the National Association of Surrogate Mothers. "[S]urrogate child-bearing is not exploitation of women," she wrote in a letter to the *New York Times*. "It is our individual right voluntarily to create a child for another family. To deprive women of this right is clearly a threat to feminist concerns."

Surrogate contracts are not an extension of the fight for women's right to control their own bodies. That fight is to secure the right of the woman to decide when and if to have children, free from interference from the government, church officials, doctors, husbands, lovers, boyfriends, or any other individuals.

This struggle has embodied the fight for birth control; sex education; safe, legal abortion; and protection from forced sterilization. It is interconnected with the broader struggle by women to be treated equally with men in all aspects of society and not be disqualified because of pregnancy, children, or lack of children.

Surrogacy contracts run completely counter to this struggle, what it has already achieved, and the future it points to. Far from an expansion of women's rights, these contracts deny rights previously conquered by women and working people as a whole.

Similar arguments to those on surrogate motherhood have been raised by some feminists about women's "right" to be prostitutes. Of course this is a degrading, antiwoman institution, they argue, but shouldn't a woman be able to sell her body if she "wants to"?

The "right" of women to sell their bodies is not the issue in prostitution—the oppression and exploitation of women is.

Prostitution involves a "contract" too. A man pays a woman for sex, and she's supposed to deliver. If she decides not to—if she "breaks" the contract—does he have a right to carry through the contract by forcibly having sex with her? No. If he tries to do that, he should be jailed for rape.

Another example is "homework"—through which textile, garment, and other employers superexploit a layer of workers. Some argue homework is okay if the workers do it "voluntarily." But the labor movement has fought long and hard against this practice, which not only denies decent wages, working conditions, and union rights to the workers directly involved, but drags down the wages and rights of all workers.

Interviews done with women who enter surrogacy contracts indicate they do so for a combination of emotional and financial reasons, all reflections of the pressures that bear down on women in this society. But whatever their motivations, the fact is that they are being brutally exploited.

And they are exploited by more than just the parties to whom they sign over their bodies for nine months. Some twenty-four surrogacy agencies now exist in this country, profiting handsomely from this traffic in women's bodies.

A *New York Times Magazine* reporter visited the offices of Noel Keane. "[H]is comfortable, two-story offices in Dearborn, Mich., were full of prospective surrogate mothers, often with husbands and babies in tow, and infertile couples who had come to check out the candidates for surrogacy," wrote reporter Anne Taylor Fleming.

"The well-groomed couples . . . were each assigned a private office, through which the surrogates were rotated, to proffer their fertility and show off the living, gurgling proof thereof."

For each woman and eventual baby he successfully markets, Keane pulls down $10,000 for himself.

Male companions of the women also get into the business. One man who accompanied his female friend to the office told Fleming, "I'll take care of her when she's pregnant again, but the baby means absolutely nothing. It's like watching someone's car for nine months. We're in it for the money; it's a business."

Keane argues that he provides a public service, that he is showing sensitivity to the "pain and cries" of the "infertile."

Judge Sorkow upheld this notion of the "rights" of the infertile. He ruled that state "refusal to enforce these [surrogate] contracts . . . would constitute an unconstitutional interference with procreative liberty since it would prevent childless couples from obtaining the means to have families."

To believe Keane and Sorkow, a new class of oppressed people—the "infertile"—has arisen. No one should deny them their "right" to "their own" child, a "right" supposedly guaranteed by the U.S. Constitution.

But Keane and Sorkow have things turned upside down.

The government has an obligation to guarantee that every *child* has protection and nurture—health care, education, and decent living conditions. This obligation extends to other dependent human beings as well, such as the aged and people who are incapacitated by physical or mental illness.

But the government has *no* obligation to guarantee every adult the "right" to "their own" child.

Judge Sorkow claims the law should recognize surrogacy contracts in order to satisfy an "intense drive to procreate." There is no instinctual drive to procreate, however. There is an instinct to have sex—procreation is sometimes a consequence.

The attitude that people must have "their" child with "their" genes so they can continue "their bloodline" or "family name" is deeply rooted in class society. William Stern presented this reactionary notion in the court case, explaining he had no living relatives because many were killed by the Nazis. He said he needed Whitehead's baby to continue "his" bloodline.

The Nazis, of course, were the most famous advocates of continuing certain bloodlines. They also ended up trying to exterminate other bloodlines they deemed socially unfit.

Under capitalism, the welfare of the child is not the principal concern nor are the rights of the woman who gives birth. Defining the line of inheritance is.

The working class, which has no property to pass on to its offspring, is nevertheless affected by ruling-class ideology about the family. Fears, insecurities, and hopes of immortality, all bred by class society, lead many working people to try to "continue the family name." This introduces enormous pressures, with the children being the greatest victims.

Surrogate mother contracts are simply the latest—and one of the most degrading—manifestations of the way capitalism treats children. If surrogacy served some socially useful purpose, it could be argued that society should promote its practice. But it serves no progressive purpose. Humanity is not on the brink of extinction. Many children are being born and many more will be. There is not a social need to increase the number of babies.

Surrogacy is not like adoption, which *is* socially necessary today. Despite the fact that adoption is immersed in profit-making and that abuses against the children and parents involved do occur, there is a need for this institution to help children without care.

This is its starting point—not the "need" of some adults to have "their" child. The concept of adoption is that society must find a way to provide care to all children lacking it. That's progressive.

The concept of surrogacy is that society owes all adults the "right" to "their" child. There's nothing progressive at all about that—it is reactionary.

It opens the door to such things as the international baby racket that has received so much publicity and condemnation. According to the *New York Times,* the number of foreign-born babies adopted in the United States shot up from 4,868 in 1981 to 9,945 in 1986. The real number is undoubtedly much higher. Most come from Asia or Latin America. Some are stolen outright from their mothers by baby dealers; others are torn away under extreme duress by these merchants.

This happens because there are fewer children in this country available for adoption than there used to be, even though racist prejudices still prevent the adoption of many U.S.-born children who are not white. Capitalist businessmen preying on couples without children see a profit to be made, because the baby "shortage" has driven the price of babies up.

But the fact that there are fewer homeless babies in the

United States is good. It marks human progress on several fronts—in relation to society's treatment of children and other human beings, the advance of science and technology, and the advance of women's rights.

In many primitive societies, when it wasn't possible to feed everybody, it was the practice to kill some infants and other dependents.

Under feudalism and lasting beyond, the first-born son in the families of the landed nobility had special rights over other children. This practice has also been wiped out.

The brutal exploitation of child labor in textile mills, coal mines, and agriculture has become illegal in this country. The labor movement won this victory, as it won the right to free, compulsory education through high school.

A century ago, many children were still losing their parents in shipwrecks, epidemics, or other events. Such children were sometimes adopted by relatives or neighbors who already had children and took in others as an elementary act of social responsibility. Often, however, they were left to fend for themselves. Today, the number of adult human beings perishing under such circumstances is greatly reduced in the United States. And children without parents generally live under much better conditions.

Social attitudes toward orphans and adopted children have also been changing in a progressive direction. These children are less often seen as somehow abnormal and deserving different treatment than children who live with a biological parent. Prejudices have also subsided with regard to children born to unmarried women—so called bastards or illegitimate children.

Humanity as a whole has advanced and deepened its solidarity for all members of society. This has been the product of struggle by workers and farmers. And it is linked to advances in science and technology that have helped working people shed various aspects of exploitation, inequality, and prejudice.

It is important to recognize the progressive role science and technology play—including under capitalism. This is especially true in light of arguments that surrogate births show society is becoming the victim of technology and predictions that science will turn most working-class women into "breeders" of babies for the rich.

The trend is actually the opposite—women are having fewer children today than ever before and they have taken giant steps away from their socially imposed role as "breeders." This has happened because of women's victories in the fight for abortion rights and birth control, changing attitudes toward women, changes in women's own self-perception, and *science*.

Scientific discoveries mean that women today are better informed about sex and health. Access to birth control and abortion, while still restricted to some degree, allows them far more decision-making power about when and if to have children. Technology has also produced labor-saving devices that have greatly reduced the hours women spend on domestic labor, further freeing them to participate in the labor force and society as a whole.

Women have seized on these advances to struggle for and win greater rights.

One result of this is a decline in the number of children women have, now that they have more freedom to plan pregnancy or decide to not have children at all. According to the U.S. Census Bureau, the average number of people per household was 2.67 in 1986, down from 3.14 in 1970.

There is also greater social acceptance of couples who live together and decide not to have children and of adults who choose to live alone, also a growing category according to the Census Bureau.

One consequence is the "shortage" of children to adopt. A new phenomenon has arisen in relation to this, that of couples frantically seeking "their own" child, frequently after not having had children earlier in life.

Technology has helped make possible the current situation where there are fewer children to adopt. Technology has benefitted women and all working people—increasing life spans, lowering infant mortality, boosting food production, and reducing labor time. And as such, it is being used by the working class to *lessen* exploitation and *reduce* class, race, and sex inequalities.

It is not technology that is responsible for abuses like surrogacy; it is capitalism, with its drive for profit and its warping of human values.

Surrogacy is and will remain a marginal practice. Far from being the "wave of the future," it is actually a throwback to the past. Judge Sorkow's ruling upholding surrogacy contracts has simply opened up the debate about this practice, exposing its real nature to many working people for the first time.

'Fathers,' 'mothers,' and rights in raising children

PUBLISHED MAY 1, 1987

My previous article on the New Jersey "Baby M" case explained that "surrogate mother" contracts are unconstitutional and therefore invalid.

To enforce such contracts is to reverse the gains conquered by the labor movement when it won the outlawing of indentured servitude. Surrogate mother contracts abuse children and violate women's rights.

Upholding such contracts also reinforces reactionary ideology about the "right" of adults to "their own" child, based on the false idea that there is an instinctual drive to procreate.

The article explained that there is no way a court can constitutionally hold Mary Beth Whitehead to the contract she signed. Under that contract, she agreed, for a $10,000 wage, to be inseminated with William Stern's sperm, to carry a pregnancy and give up her right to control her own body for nine months, and to turn over her newborn baby to Stern and his wife Elizabeth.

The March 31, 1987, court ruling—which upheld this contract, took away Whitehead's daughter Sara, and gave her to the Sterns—was reactionary. It should be reversed. The child should be allowed to live with Whitehead.

Several questions remained unanswered in that article, however, and other points were not fully developed.

Even if surrogacy contracts are invalid, wasn't the Stern-Whitehead court fight also a custody case?

Doesn't a "biological father"—the man who provides the sperm—have the same "right" to raise a child as the woman who gave birth to that child?

Doesn't a woman who provides the egg for a pregnancy have a "right" to the child even if another woman has carried the pregnancy?

The answer to all three questions is no. Let's explore the reasons why.

Judge Harvey Sorkow, who presided over the New Jersey trial, called it a "routine custody case."

His portrayal of the trial as a dispute between a "father" and a "mother" confused the issues and distracted attention from the exploitative and unjust nature of surrogacy contracts.

A custody case usually arises when two people who have been jointly raising children separate and cannot agree on who will get the children. William Stern and Mary Beth Whitehead were never jointly raising Whitehead's newborn daughter and never intended to.

Stern's sole "claim" to the child was a scrap of paper called a surrogacy contract. In upholding this "contract," the judge argued that Stern is the "biological father" of Whitehead's child. According to the judge, this gives Stern a "right" to "his own biologically genetically related child." Whitehead was merely the "surrogate" hired by Stern to "carry his child to term."

Psychologist Lee Salk, a witness called by Stern's lawyers, went so far as to propose that Whitehead be termed a "surrogate uterus" rather than a "surrogate mother," to remove any suggestion that she has a legitimate relationship to her daughter.

But it is precisely Whitehead's biological, social, and emotional relationship to the child that is key to the case. Stern's supposed "biological" connection is irrelevant.

Stern is not the "father" of Whitehead's child. Richard Whitehead, who is living with Mary Beth Whitehead and her other children, is the "father" in this case.

Being a "father" is not determined biologically (leaving aside the fact that there is no scientific way to prove it was Stern's sperm that made Whitehead pregnant).

Throughout human history, a "father" has been the husband or companion of a woman who is raising children. It is based on his relationship to the woman that a man becomes "father" to the children.

Due to death, divorce, or husbands who walk away, many women may then live with someone else, who then becomes a "father" to her children. They remain "fathers" as long as they are living with the woman and sharing responsibility for the children. In a growing number of cases, women are bringing up children without "fathers" at all.

Being a sperm donor gives no man a right to raise the resulting child, any more than being an egg donor gives a woman that right.

(In a practice called "surrogate gestation," a woman is implanted with the fertilized egg of another woman. The "surrogate gestator" carries the pregnancy and gives birth, turning the baby over to the other woman. The practice is used in some cases by a couple of one race who hire a woman of another race to bear a child who will also "look like them.")

Neither eggs nor sperm can be the basis for deciding who is the "mother" or "father" of a child, or who has the right to bring that child up. There is only one criterion that conforms to the reality of the society we live in and the obligation of society to act in the best interests of the child.

It is the woman who carries the pregnancy, gives birth to the baby, and begins nurturing that baby who has the right and responsibility to raise the child—and the right to all the social benefits she needs to do so. The only reason the state should intervene to take her child away is if she is guilty of child abuse.

Nothing of the kind was proven in the case of Mary Beth Whitehead. The Sterns brought into court an army of psychologists and social workers who insisted Whitehead was an "unfit mother." Their evidence?

Whitehead had a "narcissistic personality disorder," in part because she dyed her hair; she gave her children pandas, instead of pots and pans, to play with; she had a shouting match with a nun who teaches her son at a Catholic school; she once worked as a dancer in a bar; and her husband was an alcoholic.

Lawyers also proudly pointed out that the Sterns make more than $90,000 a year, while Whitehead is dependent on the $28,000 her husband makes as a sanitation worker.

But none of this is relevant to whether Whitehead is "unfit" to raise her child. What *is* relevant is that she gave birth to the child and began raising that child.

This applies not only in Whitehead's case, where a surrogacy contract was the key issue, but to custody cases, where a man and a woman have been living together.

Some feminists argue that men and women should have an equal "right" to child custody. Awarding the child to the woman, as the courts have generally done, is discriminatory, they say. It bolsters the false idea that women are child rearers by nature, which is used to deny them rights.

But far from advancing the struggle for women's rights, this view obscures the real issue and sets back that struggle.

We have to start with the facts. First, it is women who give birth to children. As with other mammals, the human female begins nurturing her offspring immediately after birth, feeding the child and furthering his or her development. There clearly is a natural instinct on the part of the woman to do so. And human infants have less capacity to survive on their own and require a longer period of care than other mammals.

The instinct to take care of the child one has borne is quite different from the phenomenon of wanting a child. That desire, as we pointed out in the previous article, is socially conditioned. It is not an instinct. And it does not give adults a "right" to have "their own" child.

A few women who give birth decide to put the baby up for adoption if they don't think they can provide adequate care. But that too is done as a way of seeking nurture for the infant. Only an emotionally disturbed woman reacts to her newborn child by trying to abuse or abandon the baby without any provisions for its welfare.

Moreover, as children develop, it is women who give them the greatest amount of care and nurture. This has been true since the beginning of humanity.

In today's society, if the woman is living with a man, he most likely provides financial support and may give her some help with caring for the children. He shares legal responsibility with her for the children.

But his relationship to the children, and even his sense of responsibility for them, is quite different than the woman's. If a conflict between the man and woman occurs, it's generally the man who walks away, leaving the woman and children.

The woman cannot walk away nearly so easily, especially because she faces a rougher time financially if she does so. If she does separate from the man, however, she generally takes her children with her.

All the above facts dictate that when a man and woman living together with children are separated, the burden of proof is on the *man* to show why the woman should *not* be allowed to raise the children. Unless she is proven to be abusing the children, she should get custody.

The woman's right to raise her children is not solely determined by giving birth. Take, for example, a woman who gave birth to a child five years ago and gave the baby up for adoption. Does that woman now have the right to regain custody of the child based on being the child's "real mother"?

No. There is no such thing as "mothers' rights." The issue here is women's rights and guaranteeing the best possible care for children.

In the above case, another woman has become the child's "mother." She has taken on the responsibility for the child and has the right to continue raising the child. The fact that she did not give birth to the child makes her no less "fit" to be a "mother."

And the fact that the child is adopted, not "natural," does not mean that he or she should be placed in a separate, inferior category. The child deserves the same protection and social benefits as all other children.

The very idea of "natural" vs. adopted children is only posed because for ruling-class families, the chief concern is passing on property through one's offspring. The pressures from this ruling-class outlook permeate all of society, affecting all classes.

An atmosphere is created whereby some adopted children feel compelled to search for their "real mother" or "real father."

But it is a reactionary myth that humans have an inherent drive to find out where their genes came from. It is a socially conditioned phenomenon produced by capitalism, which encourages feelings of inferiority on the part of adopted children and guilt on the part of women who put their children up for adoption.

As we discussed in the previous article, such pressures have less hold on the working class today than ever before.

In the struggle to end women's oppression and guarantee children the best care possible, the working class needs a twofold approach. It needs to fight for women's right to enter the work force and all arenas of society without any restrictions or discriminatory treatment because of their child-bearing capacities. It also needs to fight for the government to carry out its responsibility to provide care for children and all other dependent human beings, instead of allowing the burden for this care to fall on individuals, especially on women.

The government should provide low-cost child care from infancy on up. It should guarantee an education, medical care, decent housing, and recreation for all the young, aimed at helping them develop into independent human beings. All laws or practices that discriminate against children—based on class, race, sex, handicaps, or "legitimacy"—should be eliminated.

The working class must also challenge any disqualification of women based on their having or not having children. This begins with championing the right of women themselves to freely decide when and if to bear children. It means the right to safe, legal abortion and birth control, as well as sex education in the public schools. It means protection of women from forced sterilization.

Women's physical ability to bear children should not be used as a pretext to superexploit them on the job by paying them less than men, excluding them from certain jobs, or denying them employment if they are pregnant or already have children. The working class should demand equal pay for equal work and affirmative action so that women can achieve full equality in employment and education.

Workers should demand full maternity benefits for women, including the right to return to the same job—without loss of accrued seniority time—after the birth of a child. Absence from work because of pregnancy should be treated exactly like other contractual situations related to leaves from work.

For women who have children, the working class should demand all the state aid they need to care for them. And it should defend their right to have the courts compel men who walk away from shared responsibility for children to pay child support.

The struggle for these demands is part of the fight for a different type of government, one that acts in the interests of workers and farmers, not a handful of capitalist families. By bringing such a government to power, working people will lay the basis for further measures to provide care for children and to achieve equality for women.

How the 'Baby M' case relates to the working-class struggle

PUBLISHED JULY 3, 1987

The "Baby M" case has sparked a discussion among working people about society's responsibilities to children, what attitude to take toward surrogate mother contracts, who has the rights in custody cases, and how to end discrimination against women.

In my two earlier articles in the *Militant,* I argued that the judge's decision upholding the validity of the surrogacy contract and taking Mary Beth Whitehead's daughter away from her was a blow to gains the working class has won over the course of a century and a half. My starting point was where the "Baby M" case fits into the struggle of the working class to rid society of exploitation and oppression, particularly its effects on children, and our struggle to deepen human solidarity.

The *Guardian,* a radical weekly published in New York, has approached the issues in this case from an entirely different standpoint. Its view was expressed in a March 25, 1987, "Opinion & Analysis" piece by staff writer Elayne Rapping.

Rapping draws opposite conclusions to those of the *Militant* on every key point raised by this case.

The *Militant* starts from the interests of the modern working class, whose struggle against the capitalist exploiters aims to make advances in labor productivity benefit all of humanity. Gains for the working-class struggle create the best conditions for children and society's future generations.

Rapping tips her hat to what she says are the "class issues" in the case, but rapidly moves on to the "serious moral questions" raised.

From the vantage point of "morals" she demonstrates not only a failure to defend children and working people as a whole, but a betrayal of the struggle for women's rights itself, which cannot be separated from the struggle of workers and farmers to end class exploitation and all forms of oppression.

Rapping concludes that surrogacy (like prostitution), while "odious," offers "economic opportunity" to women.

She argues against Whitehead's right to raise her child, because, she says, "I am always leery of appeals to maternal instinct and 'natural law' based on biology." And in the Whitehead case, she adds, "I am particularly so. Whitehead is a woman born [!] and bred—through sex and class conditioning—to be a wife and mother and nothing more. Her identity and sense of well-being seem to depend solely upon that traditional role."

Finally, Rapping strongly sympathizes with William Stern's "right" to Whitehead's child, arguing, "Biological fatherhood, also at issue in this case, must be given its due, I think, if feminists are serious about sharing traditional female burdens as well as male privileges."

Rapping is wrong on every count. Let's review the issues in the "Baby M" case to see why.

Although the "Baby M" case is frequently presented as unusual, atypical, or highly complicated, at bottom it revolves around one simple question: Do the courts have the right to take away the child a woman bears when there is no evidence that the woman is abusing the child?

Judge Harvey Sorkow ruled yes, and backed up his decision with every antiworker and antiwoman prejudice he could scrape up—and with little regard for the protection of the child.

When Whitehead initially told the Sterns she was keeping Sara, they pounced on her doorstep with five cops and a court order from Judge Sorkow. When Whitehead then fled with Sara to Florida, the Sterns hired private detectives to chase Whitehead down and seize Sara.

William Stern argued in court that he had a "right" to the baby since he and Whitehead had signed a contract to that effect. Moreover, since his sperm (he assumed) had gone into producing the child, he was the rightful father. His lawyers argued that he deserved the infant because he needs to continue his "bloodline," since most of his relatives were murdered by the Nazis.

Even though this was not a custody case, the arguments raised by the Sterns were ones typical of ones in custody battles.

An article in the February 17, 1987, *New York Times* captured the anti-working-class and antiwoman prejudices marshaled against Whitehead in the courtroom.

"Mr. Stern," wrote the *Times,* "has appeared shy and sensitive, a biochemist who collects miniature trains and trolleys. . . .

"Years ago, he and his wife had placed their education and careers before marriage and children. The Sterns dated five years before marrying, in July 1974. Both were in their late '20s, and both had doctorates, he in biochemistry and she in human genetics."

By the time of the "Baby M" case, the article continued, William Stern was making $43,500 a year, and Elizabeth Stern, $48,000. They live in a "three-bedroom colonial home in Tenafly, a suburb of upper-middle-class professionals."

While the Sterns were getting Ph.D.s, the *Times* reporter stressed, "the Whiteheads were embarking into the rocky early years of their 13-year marriage in blue-collar towns on the Jersey Shore."

A part-time waitress who dropped out of high school, Mary Beth Whitehead had married Richard Whitehead at age sixteen. Her husband, the *Times* noted, was merely "a high school graduate, [who] became a truck driver for construction and sanitation companies, after having served 13 months on combat duty in the Mekong Delta in Vietnam."

"In late 1978," the *Times* went on, "Mr. Whitehead fell asleep at the wheel after drinking and hit three poles. He lost his drivers' license and his truck-driving job and entered Alcoholics Anonymous for a year. To help support the family, Mrs. Whitehead took a job as a dancer and bartender in her sister Beverly's bar for a few months."

The double standard employed against Mary Beth Whitehead due to her class background and sex is crystal clear. She drops out of high school, marries a Vietnam vet with a drinking problem, and winds up dancing in a bar. Even though none of these facts about her personal life bear the slightest relevance to her ability to raise children, they became the centerpiece of the Sterns' case. The goal, of course, was to paint her as a "slut" and "stupid"—"lower class," as they might say in Tenafly.

By contrast, William Stern was never asked anything in court about his personal life. Does he go to bars? Does he know any barroom dancers? Does his wife have a drinking problem?

What happened to Whitehead is common in custody cases, where the man seeks to disparage his ex-wife by charging her with extramarital sex relations or a lifestyle "unfitting" for a woman, behavior which is above question for a man. Most men in custody cases, in fact, already have a new female companion.

The Sterns' case also reeked of the anti-working-class prejudice that it's better for children to grow up in a "three-bedroom colonial home in Tenafly" than in "blue-collar towns on the Jersey Shore." Better to be raised by adults with Ph.D.s than those who wait tables or drive trucks for a living.

Rapping makes no more than a passing reference to the anti-working-class and antiwoman prejudices invoked in the courtroom. In a tone of thinly veiled contempt, she writes, "It is almost reflexive for progressive people to sympathize with the plight of Whitehead, the obvious sex and class underdog." Then she assures her readers that she, for one, will not fall prey to such "reflexes."

"[A]s feminists, we began by decrying the sole burdens of child care foisted upon us by men," she writes. "Yet, now that some men are asking to take on that burden, some of us are indignant. . . . Biological fatherhood, also at issue in this case, must be given its due, I think, if feminists are serious about sharing traditional female burdens as well as male privileges."

But is Rapping really so naive? Does she actually believe that William Stern will assume the major responsibility for raising Whitehead's daughter?

Certainly everyone in the courtroom was quite aware that Elizabeth Stern will be responsible for the child's care, not her husband. The comparisons made by the press and the Stern's lawyers made that clear. Mary Beth Whitehead, the high school dropout/go-go dancer, vs. the well-heeled

Elizabeth Stern, always referred to as "Dr. Stern"—who, after all, is more "fit" to be a mother.

In disputes between a man and woman over child custody, the issue is rarely whether he or she will raise the child better. The fight is really over which of two *women*—the former wife or the man's future wife, relative, or babysitter—will take care of the child. It's rare indeed when a man provides the sole care for a young child for any extended period of time.

But for the *child* and for working people it is better that the child remain with the woman who gave birth to it, rather than establishing a pattern of the capitalist courts reaching in and making a decision in each case based on class and sex criteria.

It is precisely on this issue—women's right and responsibility to make the decisions about raising the children they bear—that Rapping's view is most sharply at odds with that of the *Militant*.

There is something wrong with women like Whitehead who want to give birth and raise children, according to Rapping. They don't fit her utopian vision of how the world should be.

"In the socialist, feminist world we envision and work for," she says, "all men and women would have the opportunity to participate in the socialized raising of new generations, in any number of ways."

Perhaps in the society Rapping fantasizes they would. But in the society we live in and in which children grow up, they don't!

Mary Beth Whitehead, presumably, should wait until Rapping's "world" comes into being and then she can help raise children together with men in some unspecified "socialized" manner.

In the meantime, Whitehead should let the capitalist

courts take her daughter away from her, because that's the "feminist" thing to do.

"Seen in this context," Rapping continues, "Whitehead's apparently obsessive need to own and raise this infant appears in its true political light, as an expression of desperation on the part of a woman whose only self-esteem comes from her emotional involvement with her own biological offspring."

To fight for her right to raise her child is "obsessive," a sign of "desperation" on Whitehead's part. On the other hand, William and Elizabeth Stern, who used cops and private detectives to get "their" child, apparently show no signs of "desperation"; nor is William Stern's pursuit of his bloodline "obsessive."

There's no mistaking Rapping's tone. She considers Whitehead to be not only inferior to women who don't want to raise children, but inferior "morally" to middle-class and upper-class women who do. Rapping, who starts with the "serious moral questions," is no more able than anyone else to successfully place morals outside of social classes and politics. She gets rid of working-class politics and derives her values from the worst of middle-class politics and bourgeois prejudices.

Is Elizabeth Stern superior to Whitehead because she put off having children so she could become a high-paid Ph.D.?

And what if Whitehead's "only self-esteem" comes from raising her child? Does this justify the state taking her child away? Does it mean Whitehead will never develop greater self-confidence and independence and understanding of working-class politics? Does it mean that she is incapable of being changed by big new developments in the working-class movement?

Rapping seems to believe so. Whitehead, to her, is "a wife

and mother and nothing more"—exactly the stereotype of working-class women the opponents of women's liberation try to convince us is true!

Beneath the anti-working-class prejudice against Whitehead, Rapping also reveals contempt for children. There appears to be nothing more degrading, un-"feminist," and oppressive than providing care to children. But Rapping totally loses sight of the fact that it is the capitalist ruling class—not babies—that exploits and oppresses women.

And reading further, we discover that it's only *certain* women who shouldn't be raising children.

"It is interesting," says Rapping, "to compare Whitehead's emotional plight with that of the countless pregnant teens who are choosing to keep their babies because—like her—they see no other meaningful role, no other source of self-esteem, no other productive future.

"Feminists rightly deplore this trend and hope to dissuade these young women from motherhood."

But contrary to Rapping, not all feminists hold this view. Some take the correct working-class approach of helping young women who have children by fighting for child care, jobs, etc., and for a world where decisions about having children are not warped by the pressures and desperation used by capitalist oppressors and exploiters.

Whitehead's situation, Rapping continues, "is much the same. She married at 16 against her family's wishes [heaven forbid!] and began to mother. Her life's course—and its financial and emotional difficulties and traumas—were determined by that adolescent decision. Why wish her further entrenchment in that emotional and material trap?"

But were either Whitehead's supposed "financial" or "emotional difficulties" (how delicately and objectively put by Sister Rapping) determined by the fact that she gave birth while still in her teens? Is the reason that "pregnant teens"—a code word for young working-class women—are poor because they have children?

Rapping comes dangerously close here to the argument of the population-control advocates—those who tell us the poor are poor because they have too many babies. That *they* are responsible for the "financial and emotional difficulties—and traumas" of capitalist society!

The argument is a false one from start to finish. It is the standard reactionary lecture used to cover up the fact that it is capitalism, not too many babies, that is responsible for the poverty, overcrowded housing, malnutrition, and disease suffered by the great majority of the world's people. It is used to conceal the need—and real possibility—to change this by overthrowing capitalism.

Teenage women with children don't need social workers like Rapping to "deplore" their situation and "dissuade them from motherhood." They need a working-class movement that fights for the social resources necessary to give their children the best possible health care, education, and benefits. They need the right to complete their education and enter the work force with no discrimination based on the fact that they have children. They need the right to sex education, birth control, and abortion so that they—not the government or population controllers—can freely determine for themselves when and if to have children.

Women who reach reproductive age, whether or not they have children, need to become part of a living movement with a broader social purpose. They need to become part of the revolutionary communist movement and develop an understanding of their class interests. The last thing they need is a visionary middle-class sisterhood, whose members stick their noses so far up in the air when they talk about working-class women that you can hardly make out their words.

Surrogate mother contracts ruled invalid

PUBLISHED FEBRUARY 19, 1988

The New Jersey Supreme Court ruled February 3, 1988, that the surrogate mother contract in the "Baby M" case was "illegal and invalid."

The 7-to-0 ruling reversed some of the most anti-working-class aspects of the March 1987 decision by Judge Harvey Sorkow but upheld others.

Sorkow had used the power of the courts to take away the baby of Mary Beth Whitehead-Gould, against her will, and give the child to William and Elizabeth Stern. No proof was ever offered that Whitehead-Gould was unfit to raise her daughter. Sorkow's justification for his action was a surrogacy contract signed by Whitehead-Gould and William Stern.

The New Jersey Supreme Court ruling restored Whitehead-Gould as the legal mother of her child, and revoked the child's adoption by Elizabeth Stern.

However, the judges claimed that Whitehead-Gould's home is "anything but secure," and rejected her right to raise her own daughter, ordering that the girl remain with the Sterns. They did, however, grant her limited visiting rights, subject to a future court hearing, and have barred Judge Sorkow from conducting that hearing.

The New Jersey Supreme Court rejected Sorkow's argument that Whitehead-Gould must live up to the surrogacy contract because she had made an informed decision in signing it and "was not forced into the relationship." It pointed out that the surrogate mother "never makes a totally voluntary, informed decision, for quite clearly any decision before the baby's birth is, in the most important sense, uninformed, and any decision after that, compelled by a preexisting contractual commitment, the threat of a lawsuit, and the inducement of a $10,000 payment, is less than totally voluntary.

"In addition to the inducement of money," said the court, "there is the coercion of contract: the natural mother's irrevocable agreement, prior to birth, even prior to conception, to surrender the child to the adoptive couple. Such an agreement is totally unenforceable in private placement adoption. . . .

"Integral to these invalid provisions of the surrogacy contract is the related agreement, equally invalid, on the part of the natural mother to cooperate with, and not to contest, proceedings to terminate her parental rights, as well as her contractual concession, in aid of the adoption, that the child's best interests would be served by awarding custody to the natural father and his wife—all of this before she has even conceived and, in some cases, before she has the slightest idea of what the natural father and adoptive mother are like."

The court went on to argue that "this is the sale of a child, or at the very least, the sale of a mother's right to her child.

"It totally ignores the child; it takes the child from the mother regardless of her wishes and her maternal fitness."

The only surrogacy arrangement valid in New Jersey,

the court concluded, is one where no money payment is involved and where the surrogate mother is guaranteed the right to change her mind.

Thus, the judges ruled, Whitehead-Gould "is not only the natural mother, but also the legal mother, and is not to be penalized one iota because of the surrogate contract."

Having said this, however, the New Jersey Supreme Court went on to uphold Sorkow's view that this is a custody case in which William Stern has "rights" as the "father."

But it is neither a custody case nor is Stern the "father." A custody case usually arises when two people who have been jointly raising children split up and disagree over who will get the children. Whitehead-Gould and Stern never lived together nor planned to.

Stern's claim to be the "father" rests entirely on the surrogacy contract, now invalidated by the New Jersey Supreme Court, and his assertion that he is the sperm donor.

But a "father" is not defined by who claims to be the sperm donor but by whom the woman chooses to live with.

And a "father" has no "right" to raise the children of the woman who gave birth to them. It is the woman who carries the pregnancy, gives birth to the baby, and then begins to nurture that baby who has the right and responsibility to raise the child. The only legitimate reason for the state to intervene is if the woman is proven unfit to care for the child. Nothing of the kind was ever established in this case.

The New Jersey Supreme Court conceded that Whitehead-Gould was "rather harshly judged" in the original trial.

"We do not know of, and cannot conceive of, any other case where a perfectly fit mother was expected to surrender her newly born infant, perhaps forever, and was then told she was a bad mother because she did not," the judges said.

In fact, the Sterns paraded a battery of witnesses before the court who played on every anti-working-class and anti-woman prejudice common to custody cases. They stressed that the Sterns are both well-paid Ph.D. holders, which apparently places them above scrutiny, while Whitehead-Gould had once worked as a barroom dancer and was married to a sanitation worker with a drinking problem.

The New Jersey Supreme Court refused to return Whitehead-Gould's child, however. The reason: "The Sterns promise a secure home, with an understanding relationship that allows nurturing and independent growth to develop together. Mary Beth Whitehead's family life, into which Baby M would be placed, was anything but secure. . . . And today it may be even less so."

What makes it "even less so," according to the judges, is the fact that following the trial, Whitehead-Gould became pregnant by a man who was not her husband. She then divorced her husband and remarried. But this is irrelevant to her fitness to raise a child. The New Jersey Supreme Court is simply reimposing the same anti-working-class, sexual double standard used to victimize Whitehead-Gould and her daughter in the original trial.

Despite its mixed character, the New Jersey Supreme Court decision is expected to strengthen other challenges to the validity of surrogacy contracts. The Nebraska state legislature, for example, voted a few days later, 41-to-1, that such contracts are void in the state. And shortly before the New Jersey ruling, a Michigan judge ruled in a case similar to "Baby M" that surrogacy contracts are unenforceable in that state.

Women's Liberation and Socialism

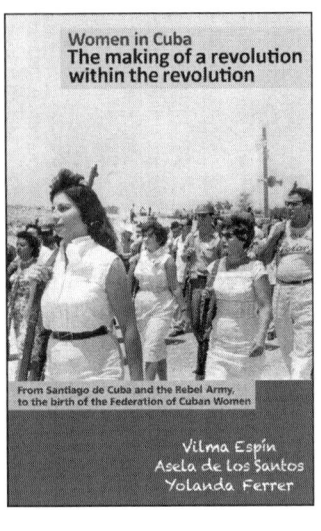

Women in Cuba: The Making of a Revolution Within the Revolution
Vilma Espín, Asela de los Santos, Yolanda Ferrer

The social revolution that in 1959 brought down the bloody Batista dictatorship began in the streets of cities like Santiago de Cuba and the Rebel Army's liberated mountain zones of eastern Cuba. The unprecedented integration of women in the ranks and leadership of this struggle was a true measure of the revolutionary course it has followed to this day. Here, in firsthand accounts by women who helped make it, is the story of that revolution—and "the revolution within." Introduction by Mary-Alice Waters. $20. Also in Spanish.

Abortion Is a Woman's Right!
Pat Grogan, Evelyn Reed

Why abortion rights are central not only to the fight for the full emancipation of women, but to forging a united and fighting labor movement. $6. Also in Spanish.

Cosmetics, Fashions, and the Exploitation of Women
Joseph Hansen, Evelyn Reed, Mary-Alice Waters

How big business plays on women's second-class status and social insecurities to market cosmetics and rake in profits. The introduction by Mary-Alice Waters explains how the entry of millions of women into the workforce during and after World War II irreversibly changed U.S. society and laid the basis for a renewed rise of struggles for women's emancipation. $15

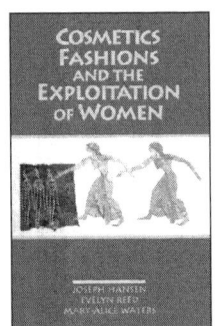

Problems of Women's Liberation
Evelyn Reed

Six articles explore the social and economic roots of women's oppression from prehistoric society to modern capitalism and point the road forward to emancipation. $15

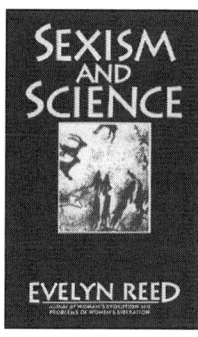

Sexism and Science
Evelyn Reed

Are human beings innately aggressive? Does biology condemn women to remain the "second sex"? Taking up such biases cloaked as the findings of science, Reed explains that the disciplines closest to human life—anthropology, biology, and sociology—are permeated with rationalizations for the oppression of women and the maintenance of the established capitalist order. $20

Women and the Family
Leon Trotsky

How the October 1917 Russian Revolution, the first victorious socialist revolution, transformed the fight for women's emancipation. Trotsky explains the Bolshevik government's steps to wipe out illiteracy, establish equality in economic and political life, set up child-care centers and public kitchens, guarantee the right to abortion and divorce, and more. $13

Communist Continuity and the Fight for Women's Liberation
Documents of the Socialist Workers Party 1971–86
Edited with an introduction by Mary-Alice Waters

How did the oppression of women begin? What class benefits? What social forces have the power to end the second-class status of women? Why is defense of a woman's right to choose abortion a pressing issue for the labor movement? This three-part series helps politically equip the generation of women and men joining battles in defense of women's rights today.
3 volumes. $30

www.pathfinderpress.com

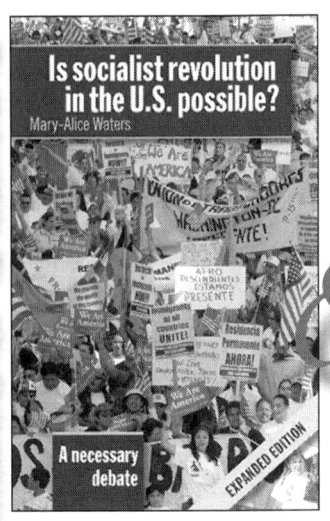 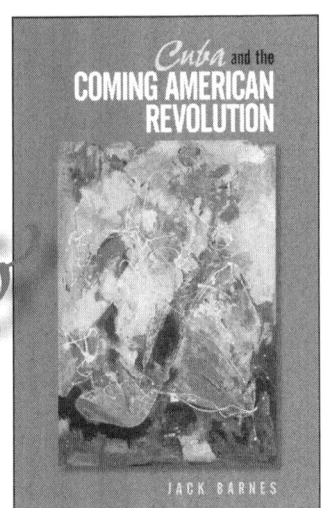

Is Socialist Revolution in the U.S. Possible?
A Necessary Debate
MARY-ALICE WATERS

In two talks, presented as part of a wide-ranging debate at the Venezuela International Book Fairs in 2007 and 2008, Waters explains why a socialist revolution in the United States is possible. Why revolutionary struggles by working people are inevitable, forced upon us by the crisis-driven assaults of the propertied classes. As solidarity grows among a fighting vanguard of working people, the outlines of coming class battles can already be seen. $7. Also in Spanish, French, and Swedish.

Cuba and the Coming American Revolution
JACK BARNES

The Cuban Revolution of 1959 had a worldwide political impact, including on working people and youth in the imperialist heartland. As the mass, proletarian-based struggle for Black rights was already advancing in the US, the social transformation fought for and won by the Cuban toilers set an example that socialist revolution is not only necessary—it can be made and defended.

This second edition, with a new foreword by Mary-Alice Waters, should be read alongside *Is Socialist Revolution in the U.S. Possible?* $10. Also in Spanish and French.

www.pathfinderpress.com

Building a PROLETARIAN PARTY

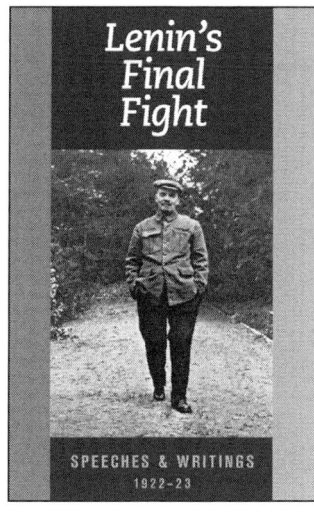

Lenin's Final Fight
Speeches and Writings, 1922–23
V.I. LENIN

In 1922 and 1923, V.I. Lenin, central leader of the world's first socialist revolution, waged what was to be his last political battle. At stake was whether that revolution, and the international movement it led, would remain on the proletarian course that had brought workers and peasants to power in October 1917. Indispensable to understanding the world class struggle in the 20th and 21st centuries. $20. Also in Spanish.

Their Trotsky and Ours
JACK BARNES

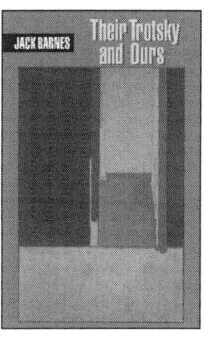

To lead the working class in a successful revolution, a mass proletarian party is needed whose cadres, well beforehand, have absorbed a world communist program, are proletarian in life and work, derive deep satisfaction from doing politics, and have forged a leadership with an acute sense of what to do next. This book is about building such a party. $16. Also in Spanish and French.

The History of American Trotskyism, 1928–38
Report of a Participant
JAMES P. CANNON

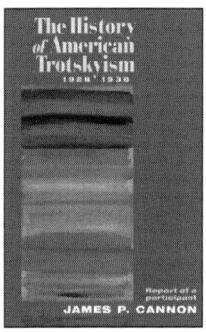

"Trotskyism is not a new movement, a new doctrine," Cannon says, "but the restoration, the revival of genuine Marxism as it was expounded and practiced in the Russian revolution and in the early days of the Communist International." In twelve talks given in 1942, Cannon recounts a decisive period in efforts to build a proletarian party in the United States. $22. Also in Spanish and French.

www.pathfinderpress.com

EXPAND *Your Revolutionary Library*

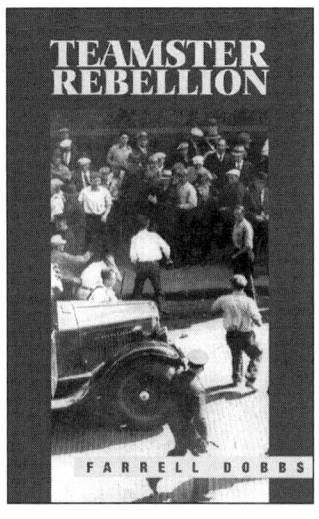

Teamster Rebellion
FARRELL DOBBS

The first of a four-volume participant's account of how strikes and organizing drives across the Midwest in the 1930s, initiated by leaders of Teamsters Local 574 in Minneapolis, paved the way for industrial unions and a fighting working-class social movement. These battles showed what workers and farmers can achieve when they have the leadership they deserve. Dobbs was a central part of that class-struggle leadership. $19. Also in Spanish, French, and Swedish.

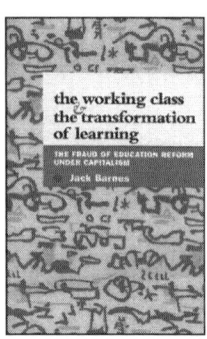

The Working Class and the Transformation of Learning
The Fraud of Education Reform under Capitalism
JACK BARNES

"Until society is reorganized so that education is a human activity from the time we are very young until the time we die, there will be no education worthy of working, creating humanity." $3. Also in Spanish, French, Swedish, Icelandic, Farsi, and Greek.

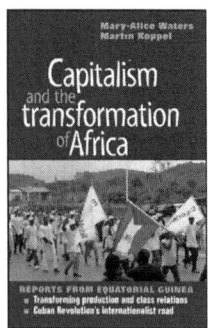

Capitalism and the Transformation of Africa
Reports from Equatorial Guinea
MARY-ALICE WATERS, MARTÍN KOPPEL

The transformation of production and class relations in a Central African country, as it is drawn deeper into the world market and both a capitalist class and modern proletariat are born. As Cuban volunteer medical brigades collaborate to transform social conditions there, the example of Cuba's socialist revolution comes alive. Woven together, the outlines of a future to be fought for today can be seen—a future in which Africa's toilers have more weight in world politics than ever before. $10. Also in Spanish.

www.pathfinderpress.com

"What Cuba can give the world is its example"
—THE SECOND DECLARATION OF HAVANA

The Cuban Five
*Who they are, Why they were framed,
Why they should be free*
MARTÍN KOPPEL, MARY-ALICE WATERS,
AND OTHERS

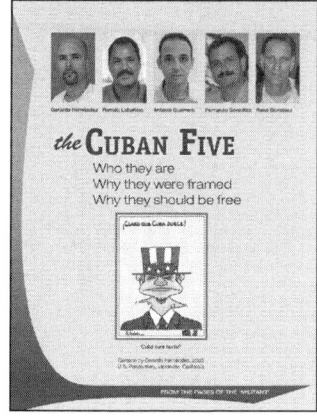

Held in US prisons since 1998, five Cuban revolutionists were framed up for being part of a "Cuban spy network" in Florida. Gerardo Hernández, Ramón Labañino, Antonio Guerrero, Fernando González, and René González were keeping tabs for the Cuban government on rightist groups with a long record of armed attacks on Cuba from US soil. Articles from the *Militant* on the truth about the frame-up and the international fight against it. $5. Also in Spanish.

Soldier of the Cuban Revolution
*From the Cane Fields of Oriente to General of the
Revolutionary Armed Forces*
LUIS ALFONSO ZAYAS

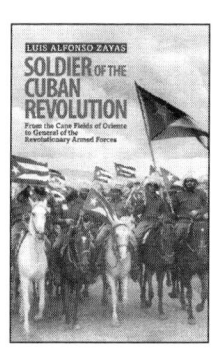

The author recounts his experiences over five decades in the revolution. From a teenage combatant in the clandestine struggle and 1956–58 war that brought down the US-backed dictatorship, to serving three times as a leader of the Cuban volunteer forces that helped Angola defeat an invasion by the army of white-supremacist South Africa, Zayas tells how he and other ordinary men and women in Cuba changed the course of history and, in the process, transformed themselves as well. $18. Also in Spanish.

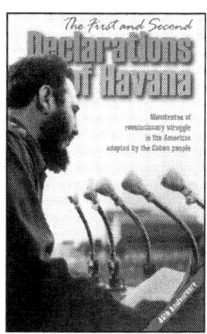

The First and Second Declarations of Havana
Nowhere are the questions of revolutionary strategy that today confront men and women on the front lines of struggles in the Americas addressed with greater truthfulness and clarity than in these uncompromising indictments of imperialist plunder and "the exploitation of man by man." Adopted by million-strong assemblies of the Cuban people in 1960 and 1962. $10. Also in Spanish, French, and Arabic.

www.pathfinderpress.com

New International
A MAGAZINE OF MARXIST POLITICS AND THEORY

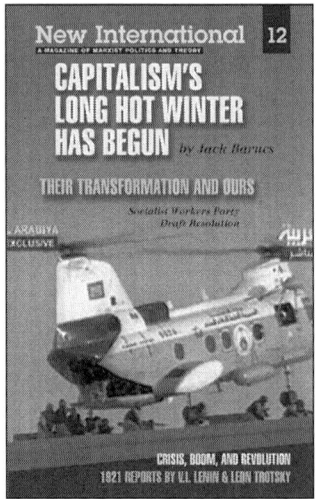

NEW INTERNATIONAL NO. 12
Capitalism's Long Hot Winter Has Begun
Jack Barnes
and *"Their Transformation and Ours,"*
Resolution of the Socialist Workers Party

Today's sharpening interimperialist conflicts are fueled both by the opening stages of what will be decades of economic, financial, and social convulsions and class battles, and by the most far-reaching shift in Washington's military policy and organization since the US buildup toward World War II. Class-struggle-minded working people must face this historic turning point for imperialism, and draw satisfaction from being "in their face" as we chart a revolutionary course to confront it. $16. Also in Spanish, French, and Swedish. *Capitalism's Long Hot Winter Has Begun* is available in Arabic.

NEW INTERNATIONAL NO. 13
Our Politics Start with the World
Jack Barnes

The huge economic and cultural inequalities between imperialist and semicolonial countries, and among classes within almost every country, are produced, reproduced, and accentuated by the workings of capitalism. For vanguard workers to build parties able to lead a successful revolutionary struggle for power in our own countries, says Jack Barnes in the lead article, our activity must be guided by a strategy to close this gap.
Also in No. 13: "Farming, Science, and the Working Classes" *by Steve Clark*. $14. Also in Spanish, French, and Swedish.

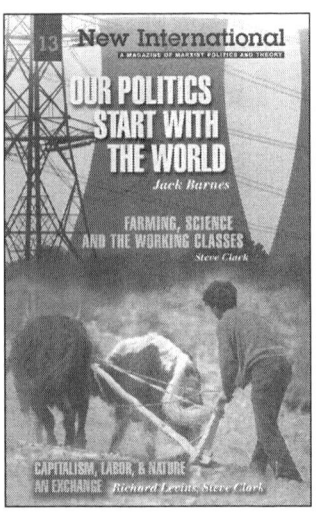

WWW.PATHFINDERPRESS.COM